About the NCCN Guidelines for Patients®

NCCN National Comprehensive Cancer Network®

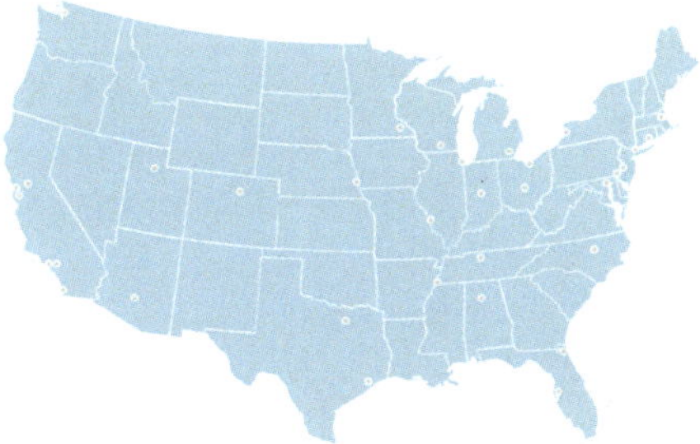

Did you know that top cancer centers across the United States work together to improve cancer care? This alliance of leading cancer centers is called the National Comprehensive Cancer Network® (NCCN®).

Cancer care is always changing. NCCN develops evidence-based cancer care recommendations used by health care providers worldwide. These frequently updated recommendations are the NCCN Clinical Practice Guidelines in Oncology (NCCN Guidelines®). The NCCN Guidelines for Patients plainly explain these expert recommendations for people with cancer and caregivers.

These NCCN Guidelines for Patients are based on the NCCN Clinical Practice Guidelines in Oncology (NCCN Guidelines®) for Management of Immunotherapy-Related Toxicities, Version 1.2024 — December 7, 2023.

View the NCCN Guidelines for Patients free online NCCN.org/patientguidelines	Find an NCCN Cancer Center near you NCCN.org/cancercenters

Connect with us

Supporters

NATIONAL COMPREHENSIVE CANCER NETWORK®
NCCN FOUNDATION
Guiding Treatment. Changing Lives.

NCCN Guidelines for Patients are supported by funding from the NCCN Foundation®

NCCN Foundation gratefully acknowledges the following corporate supporters for helping to make available these NCCN Guidelines for Patients: Bristol Myers Squibb; Kite, a Gilead Company; Pfizer Inc.; Regeneron Pharmaceuticals, Inc.; and Sanofi Genzyme.

NCCN independently adapts, updates, and hosts the NCCN Guidelines for Patients. Our corporate supporters do not participate in the development of the NCCN Guidelines for Patients and are not responsible for the content and recommendations contained therein.

To make a gift or learn more, visit online or email

NCCNFoundation.org/donate

PatientGuidelines@NCCN.org

Contents

NCCN Foundation seeks to support the millions of patients and their families affected by a cancer diagnosis by funding and distributing NCCN Guidelines for Patients. NCCN Foundation is also committed to advancing cancer treatment by funding the nation's promising doctors at the center of innovation in cancer research. For more details and the full library of patient and caregiver resources, visit NCCN.org/patients.

National Comprehensive Cancer Network (NCCN) and NCCN Foundation
3025 Chemical Road, Suite 100, Plymouth Meeting, PA 19462 USA

1
Immunotherapy basics

Immune checkpoint inhibitors have unique side effects. This guide can help you recognize possible side effects early and report them to your care team.

Overview

The possible side effects of immunotherapy range from mild to life-threatening. Doctors call them immune-related adverse events (irAEs). Most are manageable if found and treated early.

Unlike other cancer treatments, immunotherapy side effects occur because the immune system is attacking healthy cells in the body. This is similar to what happens in people with autoimmune disorders.

Reactions can start during or after immunotherapy. Some may worsen with each dose. Side effects tend to be more severe when treatment includes more than one type of checkpoint inhibitor. Main types include:

- PD-1/PD-L1 inhibitors
- CTLA-4 inhibitors
- LAG-3 inhibitors

You will be monitored for side effects and to see how treatment is working. Expect to have lab tests and physical exams on a regular basis. Tell your primary care doctor and other care providers that you are taking a checkpoint inhibitor.

Immune checkpoint inhibitors*
PD-1/PD-L1 inhibitors
cemiplimab (Libtayo) nivolumab (Opdivo) pembrolizumab (Keytruda) atezolizumab (Tecentriq) avelumab (Bavencio) durvalumab (Imfinzi) dostarlimab-gxly (Jemperli) retifanlimab-dlwr (Zynyz)
CTLA-4 inhibitors
ipilimumab (Yervoy) tremelimumab (Imjudo)
LAG-3 inhibitor
relatlimab (Opdualag)
**approved at this time*

How checkpoint inhibitors work

One job of the immune system is to spot cancerous and other abnormal cells. There are proteins on the surface of cancer cells (such as PD-L1) that interact with proteins on immune cells (such as PD-1). At these meetings, the immune cell doesn't see the cancer cell as a threat. Checkpoint inhibitors block this interaction and allow the immune cell to kill the cancer kill.

Which side effects are most common?

It is common to experience more than one side effect.
Fatigue is very common and may accompany any of the side effects.

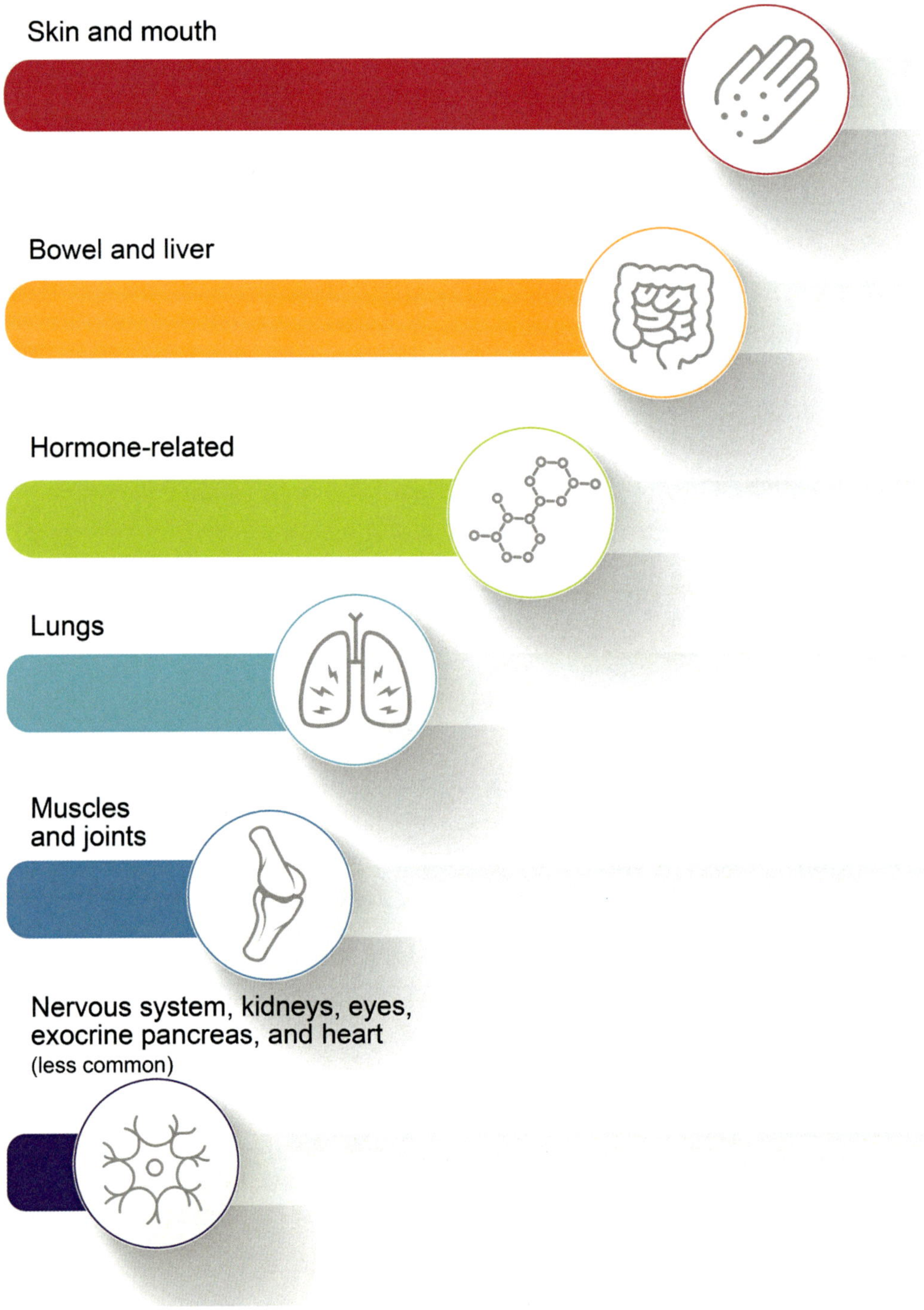

Treating side effects

Treating side effects is a team effort. Your care team will work with specialists as needed to guide your care. Some severe reactions may require treatment at a specialized care center.

In many cases, the first step in managing a side effect is to pause or discontinue immunotherapy. This should be a shared decision that you make with your provider after talking it over.

Corticosteroids

Many side effects are treated with corticosteroids (steroids for short). Steroids reduce the activity of the immune system. These are not the same as steroids used to build muscle mass (anabolic steroids). Steroids are not helpful for stopping or reversing some effects, such as hormone-related problems.

Prednisone and methylprednisolone are the most commonly used steroids. The main difference is that methylprednisolone comes in an injectable form and can be put directly into the bloodstream, rather than having to take a pill.

Steroids work best when started early. If you notice any new or worsening symptoms, don't wait to tell your care team.

Side effects

Side effects of steroid therapy include:

- Increased appetite
- Weight gain
- Mood changes
- Retaining water
- High blood pressure

Steroids can irritate the lining of the stomach. This is called gastritis. If you take other medications that also do this, your doctor may prescribe you a medication to help prevent it.

Steroids can raise blood sugar level. This is a problem for people whose blood sugar is already high due to diabetes or pre-diabetes. Blood sugar monitoring and treatment may be needed during steroid therapy.

Long-term treatment with steroids weakens the bones. This is called osteoporosis. Vitamin D and calcium can help prevent bone loss. Your doctor may also recommend physical therapy and weight-bearing exercises.

Taking steroids for a long time can also cause opportunistic infections. These are infections that are more frequent or more severe in people with weakened immune systems. Depending on the steroid dose and how long you take it, your provider may start you on an antibiotic to prevent infections.

Stopping steroids

Stopping steroids too quickly can cause anxiety, sweating, nausea, and trouble sleeping. Your care team will guide you as you lower the dose slowly, over several weeks. This is called tapering.

When steroids are not enough

Sometimes steroids are not enough and other treatments that suppress the immune system are needed. Those most often used are described next. The choice of treatment will depend on the problem and how severe it is.

Infliximab (Remicade)

Infliximab is a tumor necrosis factor (TNF) blocker. It blocks a protein in the immune system that worsens immune attack. Infliximab is given intravenously (put into the bloodstream through a vein). It can re-activate tuberculosis and the hepatitis B virus. Your blood will be tested for tuberculosis and hepatitis B and C. If you are a hepatitis carrier, you will be monitored during treatment and for a few months afterward.

Intravenous immunoglobulin therapy (IVIG)

IVIG is an IV infusion of helpful antibodies naturally made by the immune system. The antibodies (also called immunoglobulins) come from different people.

Mycophenolate mofetil (CellCept)

This oral medication slows down the immune system. It's used for a range of autoimmune problems. In people not on immunotherapy it is used to prevent rejection after an organ transplant.

Rituximab (Rituxan)

B cells are a type of immune cell that make antibodies. While most antibodies are helpful in fighting infection, sometimes B-cells make antibodies that can attack organs such as the thyroid gland. Rituximab kills B cells that have a marker called CD20. It is given by IV.

Plasmapheresis

Plasma is the watery, light yellow part of blood that contains antibodies and other proteins. In this procedure, plasma is removed from your blood and replaced with plasma from a donor. It is also called plasma exchange.

Methotrexate

Methotrexate is a type of medicine called an antimetabolite. It slows down the body's immune system. In people not on immunotherapy, methotrexate is used most often to treat inflammatory conditions (such as rheumatoid arthritis) and some cancers.

After a severe side effect

Immunotherapy may be paused for certain severe side effects. Restarting treatment with the same checkpoint inhibitor isn't always possible. This may be the case even for less severe effects.

If you have the option of resuming your checkpoint inhibitor after a severe side effect, you will want to make an informed decision. Discuss the benefits and harms with your care team. If other cancer treatment is working, it may not make sense to restart immunotherapy. The anti-cancer benefits may not be worth the risk of another severe problem.

Communication is key

Stay in close contact with your care team, especially the nurses. While many side effects come on slowly, others can start and worsen quickly. Reporting symptoms when they start can help find problems early. It also helps prevent severe complications. Symptoms that seem unrelated, like diarrhea and shortness of breath, could be signs of an irAE.

If you need to go on steroids, the process of tapering (slowly stopping) takes 4 to 6 weeks, sometimes longer. During this time you will be in close contact with your care team to monitor your dose. The dose changes will be noted in your record. This is important information used to guide your care.

Ask your care team if there is a way to report your symptoms online. Patient portals or messaging systems can be an easy way to communicate with your team. However, new or worsening side effects may need urgent attention. Be sure to contact your care team using the most efficient method.

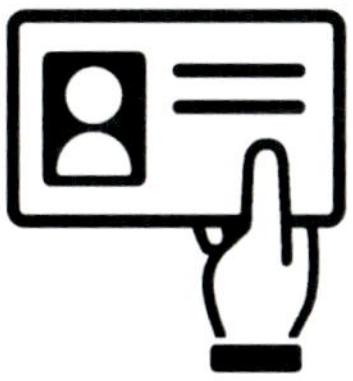

Immunotherapy Wallet Card

Ask your care team for an immunotherapy wallet card. This card lists your immunotherapy regimen, potential side effects, and contact numbers for your cancer care team. Carry it with you at all times. If a card is not available, ask for a printable list of your treatment regimen.

A printable card is available from the Oncology Nursing Society (ONS) website.

Key points

- Immunotherapy uses the immune system to kill cancer cells.
- Immune checkpoint inhibitors cause immune cells to attack cancer cells. Sometimes they also attack healthy cells. This causes side effects called immune-related adverse events (irAEs).
- Most side effects are treated with steroids (prednisone or methylprednisolone).
- Side effects of steroids include increased hunger, weight gain, mood changes, retaining water, and high blood pressure.
- Steroids are stopped by slowly lowering the dose over 4 to 6 weeks. This is called tapering.
- Other immune-suppressing treatments may be needed for side effects that do not improve with steroids.
- Stay in close contact with your care team. Ask if you can contact them online using a patient portal or messaging system.

"Check point inhibitors can have some pretty serious side effects. My husband had some really awful ones. But when these drugs work, they really work. When I asked him if he'd do it again if needed, his response was 'in a heartbeat!'"

2
Skin and mouth

Skin problems are common during treatment with a checkpoint inhibitor. Most are mild and can be managed without stopping immunotherapy. While rare, very serious skin reactions can occur.

Skin

Immunotherapy-related skin issues usually start in the first few weeks of treatment. If you develop symptoms of a skin problem, your doctor will do a full-body skin exam. This includes:

- The inside of the mouth
- Hair and scalp
- Fingernails and toenails

The goal is to find all problem areas and learn how much of the body is affected. Your provider may take pictures of the problem areas to track healing. If you have a history of skin problems, tell your care team. In this case, seeing a dermatologist on a regular basis is recommended.

Your provider will ask about your symptoms and how much they are affecting your normal activities and self-care. They may order blood testing for a severe drug reaction syndrome that causes fever, rash, and swelling of the face and hands. Depending on your symptoms, a small piece of tissue may be removed for testing (a skin biopsy).

Rash

A rash that has both flat patches and bumps is common during immunotherapy. Doctors call this a maculopapular rash. It often starts in the area between the hips and shoulders (the torso) and grows outward. You might also have other symptoms like itching, burning, or tightness. Blistering rashes are more serious than maculopapular rashes and should be reported to your care team right away (see next page).

Using an emollient is recommended for everyone with a rash. These ingredients found in skin care products soothe, moisturize, and protect the skin from irritation. They are also called barrier creams.

For a rash affecting a small area (less than 30 percent) of the body, immunotherapy can be continued. You will be prescribed a topical steroid to apply at home. Topical means it is applied to the top of the skin. It could be a cream, ointment, lotion, or gel. If the rash is itchy, your doctor may prescribe an oral antihistamine to see if it helps relieve the itching.

A rash covering more than 30 percent of the body that is interfering with basic self-care, such as bathing, is considered severe. Immunotherapy will be paused. Your doctor will consult with a dermatologist right away. In-hospital care may be needed. A tiny piece of inflamed skin may be removed and tested (a biopsy). Treatment with both a topical steroid and systemic (oral or intravenous) steroids is recommended.

Blisters

A blister is a fluid-filled sac in the outer layer of skin. Blistering is a medical emergency, especially when it affects the mouth or genitals. It may be a sign of a rare and serious disorder in which the outer layer of skin separates from the connective tissue beneath it. Your doctor will consult with a skin expert (dermatologist) right away.

The contents of an unbroken blister are usually removed and tested. It is also common to have blood tests to look for specific antibodies (proteins).

For blistering in one small area with no other symptoms, your doctor will prescribe a high-strength topical steroid. It should be applied to all inflamed and blistered areas. Immunotherapy may be paused until all blisters have healed.

For blistering affecting a larger area of the body, immunotherapy will be paused. Treatment with systemic (oral or IV) steroids will be started. If there is no improvement, your doctor may add treatment with rituximab (Rituxan) or dupilumab (Dupixent). Intravenous immunoglobulin (IVIG) may be given with either of these for severe blistering. In-hospital care is needed for severe or life-threatening blistering. Immunotherapy will be stopped.

Itching

Itching (pruritus) is also common, with or without a rash. The itching may be constant or may come and go. Oral antihistamines (allergy medicines) are recommended to help lessen itching. Using a fragrance-free moisturizer all over the body can also help relieve and prevent itching.

For mild itching in a small area, you will be prescribed a medium-strength topical steroid. Your provider may also suggest an over-the-counter pain and itch relief cream.

Itching is common during immunotherapy. Treatment with a topical steroid is recommended for mild and moderate rashes. An oral antihistamine can help relieve the itching.

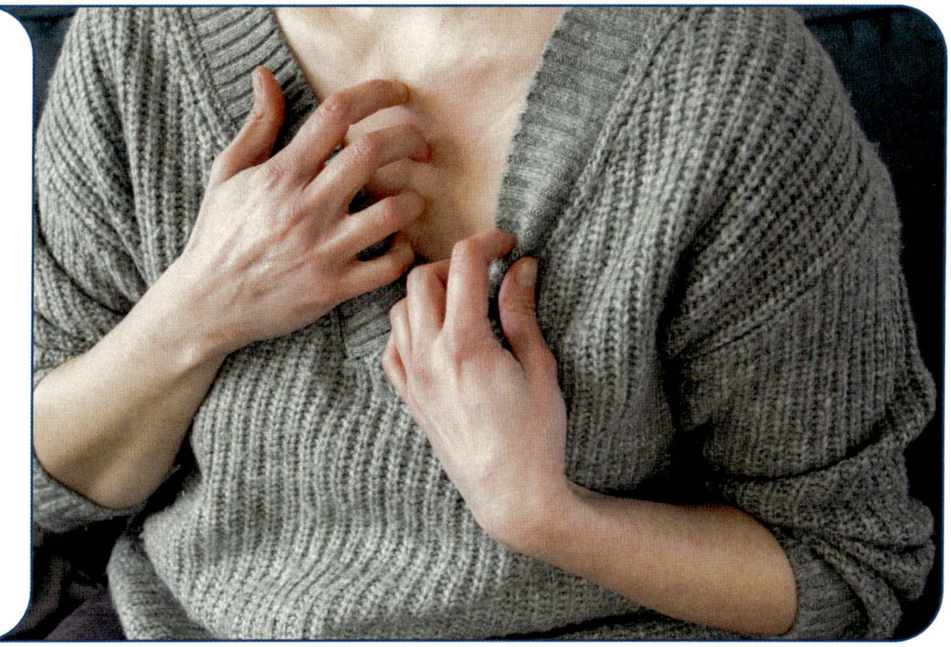

More intense or widespread itching that comes and goes is considered moderate. There are often skin changes from picking and scratching, such as lesions, bumps, swelling, oozing, crusting, or thickening of the skin. Your provider will prescribe a high-strength topical steroid. Immunotherapy will be paused until there is improvement. They may also prescribe gabapentin or pregabalin. These oral drugs can help relieve itching. If there is no improvement, light therapy (called narrow-band ultraviolet B [UVB] phototherapy) will be considered.

For itching that is constant and intense or widespread, immunotherapy will be paused. Treatment with systemic (oral or IV) steroids will be started. Your provider may also prescribe gabapentin or pregabalin. If there is no improvement in about a month, you may be prescribed dupilumab (Dupixent). This is a biologic medicine given under the skin by injection.

Lichen planus

Lichen planus is a condition that can affect the skin on the body or the inside of the mouth. On the skin it causes reddish-purple bumps and patches that are usually itchy. Inside the mouth it causes erosions (shallow indents) in mouth tissue. Intersecting fine white lines and dots can often be seen.

Treatment with either a tacrolimus-based ointment or a high-strength topical steroid is recommended. The steroid is often a gel for the mouth, a solution for the scalp, and a cream, lotion, or ointment for other affected areas.

Depending on how much of the body is affected, treatment with a systemic (oral or IV) steroid may also be needed. For severe lichen planus covering more than 30 percent of the body, your doctor will also consider treatment with other types of anti-inflammatory medicines. If available, your provider may recommend narrow-band ultraviolet B (UVB) light therapy.

Psoriasis and related diseases

Psoriasis shows up as thick, red, and scaly patches on the skin. It occurs most often in the following areas:

- Around the joints
- On the scalp
- Around the navel (belly button)
- Behind the ears

If only a small area of the body (less than 10 percent) is affected, immunotherapy can usually be continued. Your doctor will prescribe a high-strength topical steroid and a vitamin D cream or ointment, such as calcipotriene.

If a larger area of the body is affected, immunotherapy will be paused. You will start treatment with a high-strength topical steroid and a vitamin D cream or ointment, such as calcipotriene. Treatment with one of the following may be added:

- apremilast (Otezla)
- acitretin (not for people of childbearing age)
- cyclosporine
- methotrexate

You will be referred to a dermatologist to see if treatment with a biologic is an option. These protein-based drugs target specific parts of the immune system. Biologics are made in a lab from living cells. They are given by injection or through a vein.

If available, narrow-band UVB light therapy may also help with moderate or severe psoriasis.

UVB light therapy

Narrow-band UVB light therapy may help improve psoriasis or lichen planus that hasn't responded to other treatment.

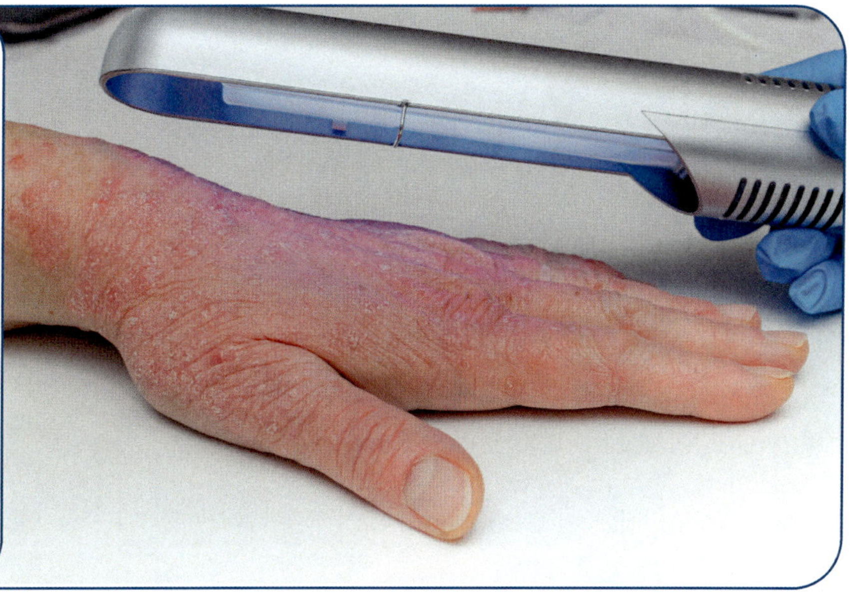

Mouth

The moist, inner lining of the mouth is called the (oral) mucosa. Symptoms can include:

- Dry mouth
- Mouth pain
- Irritated mouth, gums, and/or throat
- Mouth sores or blisters
- Changes in mouth tissue
- Sensitive gums or teeth
- Changes in taste

Your provider will examine your mucosa, gums, jaw, tongue, and teeth. They will ask about your symptoms, and whether you've had to change what you normally eat and drink.

Your doctor may remove a small piece of tissue from your lip or inside your mouth. They may also use a cotton swab to collect samples from areas of concern. The sample will be tested for fungal and viral infections.

Depending on your symptoms, making changes to your diet may help. Avoid crunchy, spicy, acidic, or hot food/drinks as needed for comfort.

Try to maintain good oral hygiene. An oral rinse that contains chlorhexidine is recommended. This medicine kills or prevents the growth of bacteria in your mouth. It also reduces swelling and irritation of the gums.

If available, your doctor may refer you to a specialist. This could be a dermatologist, oral medicine specialist, dentist, or ear, nose, and throat (ENT) doctor.

Inflamed mucosa

Immunotherapy can cause your mouth to become sore and inflamed. Symptoms of an inflamed mucosa include irritated gums or throat, mouth sores, and lichen planus. Lichen planus is described earlier in this chapter.

If you only have some food restrictions, your symptoms are considered mild. You can continue immunotherapy. Reducing the amount of acid your stomach makes can help. Treatment with a proton pump inhibitor (PPI) or a histamine-2 (H2) blocker is recommended.

You will also be prescribed a high-strength topical steroid. This may be a liquid that you swish around your mouth, or a gel applied to affected areas. Magic mouthwash can also help. This mouth rinse is a mixture of 3 things:

- An anesthetic (relieves pain)
- An antihistamine (relieves inflammation)
- An antacid (helps the other ingredients coat the mouth)

For more severe symptoms, immunotherapy will be paused. Treatment with both a topical and systemic (oral or IV) steroids is needed. If you can't eat at all, you will be admitted to the hospital.

Dry mouth

Also called sicca syndrome, dry mouth is common during immunotherapy. It's caused by the immune system attacking the glands that make saliva. Steroids may help a little, but long-term care for the lack of saliva is usually needed.

Blood tests for specific antibodies (proteins) can help diagnose sicca syndrome. Your provider will also check to see if you're taking any medicines that worsen dry mouth.

If your symptoms are mild and you don't need to change your normal eating habits much, you can continue immunotherapy. Try to drink more fluids and limit caffeine intake. Even taking small sips of water throughout the day can help.

Saliva substitutes and moisture-preserving mouth rinses, toothpastes, and sprays are recommended. Sugarless chewing gum, lozenges, or candy can also help your mouth make more saliva.

For more severe symptoms, immunotherapy will be paused. Treatment with an oral steroid will be started. Your doctor will also prescribe a cholinergic agonist. These are oral medicines that increase the amount of saliva in the mouth. If you are unable to eat at all, you will be admitted to the hospital.

Saliva protects your teeth. Not making enough saliva can lead to cavities and tooth loss. Your doctor may refer you to a dental health specialist to help avoid these problems.

Mouth pain

Mouth pain is also possible during immunotherapy. It is often described as a burning feeling. It may occur alone or with other symptoms. People often report that the pain seems worse than it should given any other symptoms.

Your care team will rule out other possible causes of the pain. They will check for problems of the jaw and/or teeth, such as an infection or abnormal growth. They will also inspect the tongue and all of the skin inside the mouth.

Treatment with a topical steroid is one option. This will likely be a gel, a dental paste, or an elixir that you swish and hold in the mouth. Viscous lidocaine is another option. This numbing mouth rinse helps relieve pain and swelling in the mouth and throat.

If the pain is mild and isn't affecting your eating or drinking habits, you can continue immunotherapy. For more severe symptoms, immunotherapy will be paused. Your doctor will also consider treatment with gabapentin.

Key points

- Skin reactions to immunotherapy can include rash, itching, blisters (rare), lichen planus, and psoriasis.
- Most skin reactions are mild and can be treated with a topical steroid. This could be a cream, ointment, lotion, gel, or foam.
- For more severe skin symptoms, systemic (oral or intravenous) steroids are needed.
- Immunotherapy can cause your mouth, gums, and/or throat to become sore and irritated.
- Other possible symptoms include dry mouth, pain or burning, sores, changes in mouth tissue, and changes in taste.
- Depending on your symptoms, avoiding crunchy, spicy, acidic, or hot food/drinks may help.
- An oral rinse that contains chlorhexidine can help prevent the growth of bacteria in your mouth and reduce gum irritation.

3

Fatigue

Feeling tired is common during immunotherapy. It can often be managed without stopping treatment. Severe fatigue, however, can be a sign of a heart or hormone problem. Urgent testing and treatment may be needed.

Testing

Your doctor will want to check some things if you have fatigue. Blood tests, a physical exam, and a check of your medications are recommended. Blood tests ordered for fatigue are listed in **Guide 1.**

Fatigue can cause or worsen depression. Expect your provider to ask about your mental health and whether you are feeling depressed.

Tell your care team about all the medications you are taking. This includes prescription and over-the-counter drugs. They may make changes to the types or doses to see if it helps.

Guide 1
Blood tests used to evaluate fatigue

General health tests	• Complete blood count (CBC) • Comprehensive metabolic panel (CMP)
Hormone tests	• Thyroid-stimulating hormone (TSH) • Free thyroxine (T4) • Cortisol • Adrenocorticotropic hormone (ACTH) • Testosterone
Heart enzyme tests	• Creatine kinase • Myoglobin • Troponin

Treatment

Fatigue can be an early sign of a severe side effect. If this has been ruled out, lifestyle changes may help. They include:

- Physical activity
- Practicing good sleep habits
- Making changes to your diet
- Staying hydrated

If your fatigue doesn't get better after resting, you and your care team will make a plan for managing it. They will look for any treatable causes of your symptoms. If none are found, you may be prescribed a low-dose oral steroid. Immunotherapy may be paused to see if there is improvement. Tell your team if your fatigue gets worse or if you notice other health issues.

For severe fatigue that is preventing basic self-care, immunotherapy will be paused or stopped. Your doctor will consider other possible causes, such as the cancer worsening or an unknown health problem. Any treatable causes will be managed.

For more information, see the *NCCN Guidelines for Patients: Fatigue and Cancer* at NCCN.org/patientguidelines and on the NCCN Patient Guides for Cancer app.

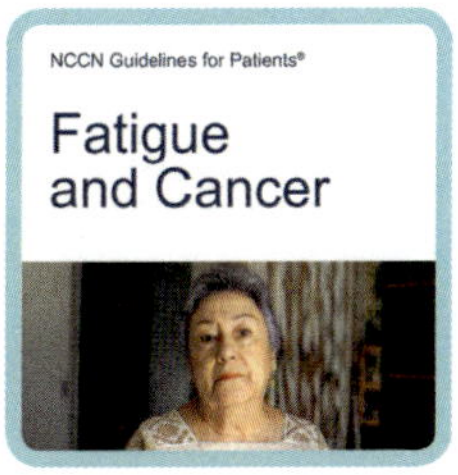

Key points

- Fatigue (tiredness) is a common side effect of immune checkpoint inhibitors.
- Severe fatigue could be a sign of a hormone problem. Urgent testing and treatment may be needed.
- Fatigue can be an early sign of a heart problem. Prompt evaluation can prevent severe complications. Hospitalization may be needed if a heart problem is found.
- Evaluating fatigue includes a physical exam, blood tests, and a medication review.
- Your doctor may make changes to your medications to see if it lessens your fatigue.
- Lifestyle changes can help with fatigue. Hydration, diet changes, and practicing good sleep habits are recommended.
- Immunotherapy can be continued for mild fatigue but may be paused if it becomes more severe.

4

Bowel and liver

Immune checkpoint inhibitors often cause diarrhea and other bowel problems. Symptoms typically start in the first 6 to 8 weeks of treatment. The liver can also become inflamed, but this does not typically cause symptoms.

Diarrhea and inflamed bowel

Diarrhea, or having more bowel movements than usual, is common during immunotherapy. The lining of the colon (large bowel) can also become inflamed. This is called colitis. Symptoms include:

- Watery stools
- Cramping
- Urgency
- Abdominal pain
- Blood (if severe) or mucus in stool
- Fever
- Nighttime bowel movements

Everyone's baseline (starting) bowel habits are different before immunotherapy. It's good to know yours, as it is often the changes in your habits that are important. Knowing how often you have a bowel movement (per day or every 1 to 2 days) and the consistency of your bowel movements can help you know what your baseline bowel pattern looks like.

Testing

Your doctor may want to test your stool (poop). The goal is to rule out infection as the cause of your symptoms. Testing will look for bacteria, viruses, and sometimes parasites. Your stool may also be tested for proteins found in stool when the bowel is inflamed.

For more severe symptoms, testing may include imaging of your abdomen and pelvis. Procedures to see inside the bowel, esophagus, and stomach may also be needed.

Treatment

Depending on your baseline habits, mild symptoms may mean 1 to 3 bowel movements above normal per day and no colitis symptoms. Anti-diarrheal medications can help. Try to drink more fluids than usual. If needed, your doctor may prescribe mesalamine and/or cholestyramine. Mesalamine is an anti-inflammatory drug taken by mouth. Cholestyramine is most often used to lower cholesterol but can also relieve diarrhea. Try to avoid foods with lactose. A BRAT (bananas, rice, apple sauce, toast) diet may help make stools firmer and less frequent.

Immunotherapy is usually paused for more severe symptoms. Depending on your starting habits, this could mean at least 4 bowel movements above normal per day along with colitis symptoms. Treatment with systemic (oral or intravenous) steroids is needed. If there is no improvement, an infusion of infliximab (Remicade) or vedolizumab (Entyvio) may be given. Based on the response, you may receive additional doses. If these treatments don't help, other immune-suppressing drugs will be considered.

Hepatitis

The liver is a large organ located on the right side of the body, under the rib cage. It filters blood and helps digest food by making a substance called bile.

The levels of substances (enzymes) made by the liver will be checked using blood tests. High levels may be a sign that the liver is inflamed or damaged. This is called hepatitis. It doesn't usually cause symptoms.

Some drugs can damage the liver. Taking too much acetaminophen (Tylenol), for example, can cause liver injury. Certain dietary supplements and alcohol use can also damage the liver. Your doctor will review all of your medications and supplements. Use of drugs that may harm the liver will be avoided or limited. Others will be adjusted based on how well your liver is working.

If liver enzyme levels get too high, treatment with steroids is needed. Immunotherapy may be paused. If there is no improvement, mycophenolate mofetil may be added. It is an immune-suppressing drug.

Bilirubin is a yellow substance in blood. Liver problems can cause it to build up in blood. If bilirubin and liver enzyme levels are very high, liver failure could occur. In-hospital care is needed.

Key points

- Diarrhea and inflamed bowel (colitis) are common side effects of immunotherapy.
- Diarrhea is an increase in bowel movements, which may be watery.
- Symptoms of inflamed bowel include watery stools, bleeding, mucus, cramping, urgency, abdominal pain, and fever.
- Anti-diarrheal medication and staying hydrated can help relieve mild symptoms. Avoiding lactose and/or starting a BRAT diet may make stools firmer and less frequent.
- Mesalamine or cholestyramine may be added for mild symptoms that don't improve with anti-diarrheal medication.
- More severe bowel symptoms are treated with steroids. Infliximab or vedolizumab may be added if needed.
- Immunotherapy can cause the liver to become inflamed (hepatitis). This doesn't usually cause symptoms. If liver enzyme levels become too high, treatment with steroids is needed.

5
Hormones

Immune checkpoint inhibitors can affect organs and glands that make hormones. Hormone-related side effects are fairly common. They are also usually permanent. Stopping immunotherapy does not reverse these side effects.

Hormones are substances that travel in blood. They regulate many important body functions.

Thyroid

The thyroid is a gland in the neck. It makes the hormones thyroxine (T4) and triiodothyronine (T3). Together they are often called just "thyroid hormone." Thyroid hormone helps many organs function properly (such as your heart and gut) and helps regulate metabolism and body temperature. Thyroid hormone levels will be checked with blood tests before and during immunotherapy.

Thyroiditis

Painless irritation of the thyroid gland caused by immune system attack is called thyroiditis. First, hormone levels rise. This doesn't usually cause symptoms. If it does, you may have weight loss, fatigue, sweating, or anxiety. If you have symptoms, your doctor may prescribe a beta-blocker. This type of drug blocks the effects of stress hormones on the heart.

After 4 to 6 weeks, thyroid hormone levels may drop, but may also return to normal.

Sometimes the level drops too low. This is hypothyroidism or underactive thyroid. Symptoms include:

- Weight gain
- Constipation
- Dry skin
- Sensitivity to the cold

You will be prescribed a medicine that replaces thyroid hormone. It is called levothyroxine. It is taken as a pill once a day. Determining the right dose for you can take some trial and error.

Pituitary

The pituitary is a gland in the brain. It makes hormones that control other glands and body functions. If the pituitary becomes inflamed, it does not make enough of certain hormones. The problems that can result are described below. Permanent damage to the pituitary can occur.

Testing for pituitary problems includes blood tests and sometimes magnetic resonance imaging (MRI) of the brain.

Secondary adrenal insufficiency

This condition occurs when the pituitary doesn't make enough adrenocorticotropic hormone (ACTH). As a result, glands on top of the kidneys (adrenal glands) do not make enough cortisol. Cortisol helps the body respond to stress, fight infection, and regulate blood sugar. The most common symptoms of low cortisol due to pituitary damage include:

- Fatigue
- Loss of appetite
- Muscle weakness

Secondary adrenal insufficiency is managed with medication to replace the hormones not being made by the body. This includes hydrocortisone tablets to replace natural cortisol. They may be needed for the rest of your life. Your doctor will determine the lowest dose needed to prevent symptoms.

Normally, the adrenal glands make much more cortisol at certain times. This happens when there is infection, illness, injury, or trauma to the body. In these cases your dose of hormone replacement therapy may be temporarily increased. Wearing a medical alert bracelet is recommended for this pituitary problem.

Rarely, the level of cortisol can become dangerously low. This is known as an adrenal crisis. In-hospital care is needed. Symptoms of adrenal crisis are listed in **Guide 2.**

Central hypothyroidism

This is a rare form of underactive thyroid. In this type the level of thyroid hormone is too low due to a problem with the pituitary or hypothalamus. The symptoms are the same as those normally seen with underactive thyroid. Weight gain, constipation, dry skin, and sensitivity to cold are most common. Your doctor will prescribe levothyroxine. This medication replaces thyroid hormone.

Guide 2 Adrenal crisis symptoms
Severe fatigue
Nausea/vomiting
Low blood pressure
Confusion
Feeling sleepy or tired
Headache*
Increased sensitivity to light*
Vision changes*
**Less common*

Pancreas

The pancreas is a gland behind the stomach. One of its jobs is to make a hormone called insulin. Insulin absorbs glucose (sugar) into cells for use as energy. If the pancreas becomes inflamed or damaged, it does not make enough insulin. This is type 1 diabetes. It is a rare side effect of immunotherapy.

Type 1 diabetes requires daily insulin therapy for life. Living with diabetes can be hard but managing it has come a long way. There are new ways to monitor and manage blood sugar. Many people find continuous glucose monitors (CGM) to be an easy way to check blood sugar.

Blood tests are used to monitor for type 1 diabetes. Your blood sugar level will be checked each time you receive immunotherapy. Further testing will be ordered if the blood sugar level is too high. Testing is also needed if you have symptoms of a diabetic emergency, described next.

Diabetic ketoacidosis

Diabetic ketoacidosis (DKA) is a blood sugar crisis. It occurs when blood sugar becomes very high. Fat is broken down too quickly and toxic acids build up in the blood and urine. It can be life-threatening if insulin is not received. Symptoms of diabetic ketoacidosis include:

- Vomiting
- Confusion
- Abdominal pain
- Fast heart beat
- Fruity odor on the breath

If you have any of these symptoms, tell your care team right away.

The pancreas

The pancreas is a large gland behind the stomach. During immunotherapy the immune system can attack the pancreas. This causes damage that affects hormone levels.

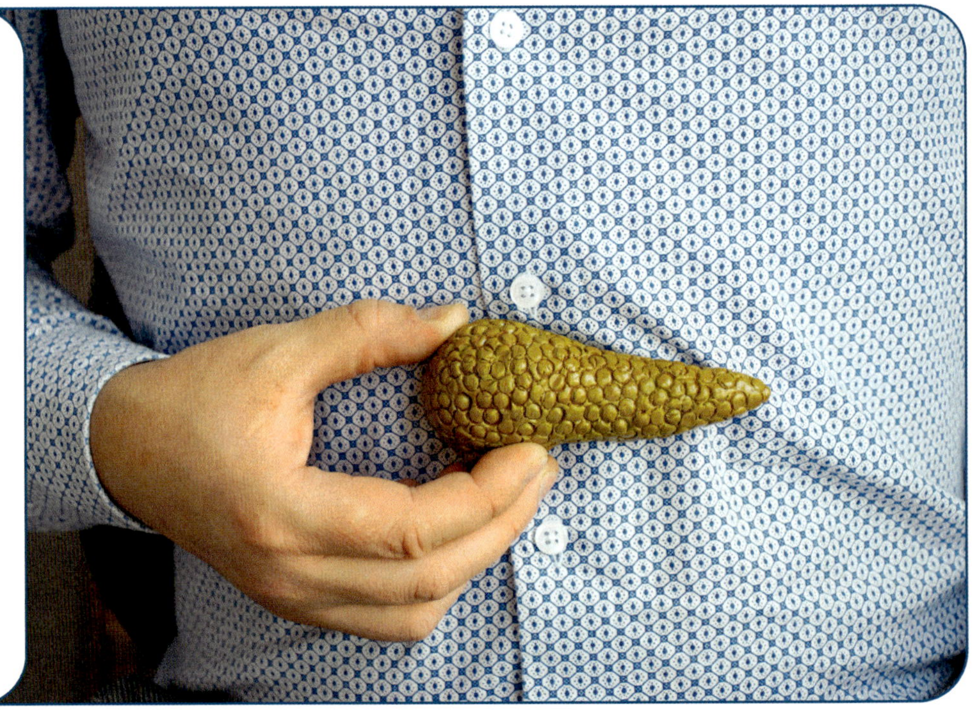

Key points

- The thyroid, pituitary, and/or pancreas may become inflamed during immunotherapy. The damage disrupts hormone levels and causes health problems that are usually permanent. Stopping immunotherapy does not reverse them.
- Thyroiditis is painless damage to the thyroid gland. Thyroid hormone levels often rise before dropping too low, causing symptoms such as weight gain, dry skin, and constipation. A medicine that replaces thyroid hormone is used to treat underactive thyroid.
- Symptoms of low cortisol due to pituitary damage include fatigue, loss of appetite, and muscle weakness. It is treated with hydrocortisone tablets. An adrenal crisis can occur if cortisol gets very low. Symptoms include severe fatigue, nausea/vomiting, and headache.
- Type 1 diabetes is a rare side effect that requires lifelong treatment with insulin. A diabetic emergency can occur if blood sugar becomes too high. Symptoms include vomiting, confusion, abdominal pain, and fast heart beat.

"If it weren't for cancer, I'd say I had the perfect life. If it weren't for cancer, would I even realize this?"

6
Lungs

The lungs can become inflamed during immunotherapy. This is called pneumonitis. The most common symptom is trouble breathing. Other symptoms include dry (mucus-free) cough, fever, chest pain, and low oxygen levels. Pneumonitis can be seen on imaging tests, even in those without symptoms.

Testing

The first sign of pneumonitis is often a low level of oxygen in the blood. In addition to a physical exam, you will have a fast and painless oxygen saturation test. This is done using a small device called a pulse oximeter placed on your fingertip. The level will be checked when you are at rest and after moving.

Computed tomography (CT)

A CT scan of your chest will likely be ordered to rule out other causes of your symptoms. If so, a liquid called a contrast agent will be used. It is typically put directly into your bloodstream through a vein to help make the CT images clearer.

Ruling out infection

It can be helpful to rule out infection as the cause of pneumonitis, especially in more

Checking your blood oxygen level

A pulse oximeter measures the amount of oxygen being carried by red blood cells. It does this by shining light through your finger.

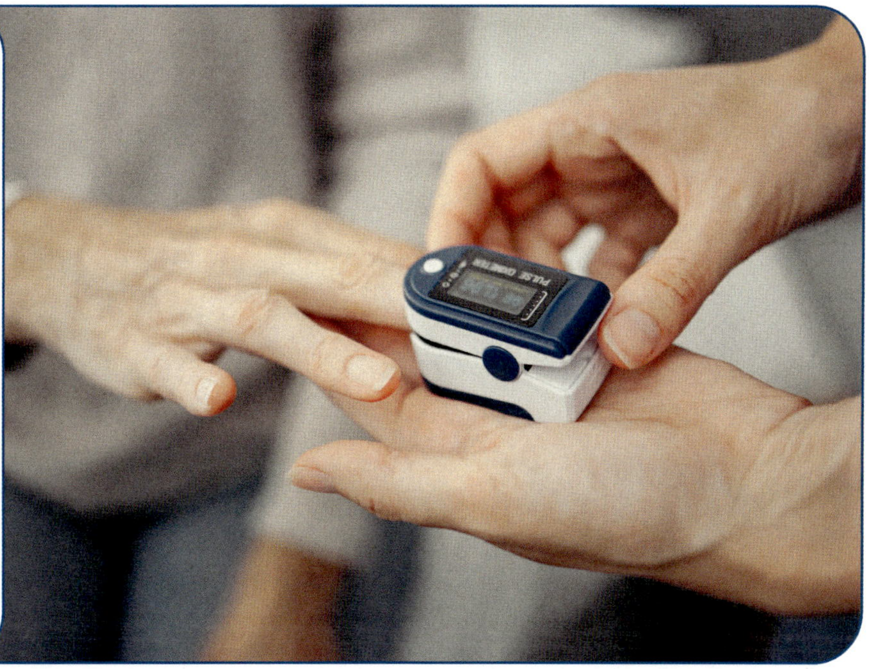

severe cases. Your provider is likely to swab the inside of your nose to detect viruses, such as the flu and COVID-19. They may also order tests of your phlegm (mucus), blood, and urine.

Another test that can help rule out infection is bronchoscopy. This minimally invasive procedure allows your doctor to see inside your lungs. A thin, flexible camera with a tiny light is guided through your nose or mouth and into your lungs. A small amount of sterile saline (saltwater) is flushed through the tube to rinse a small part of your lungs. The saline is then suctioned back through the tube and sent to a lab for testing. This is called a bronchoalveolar lavage. It is typically done with some medicine to make you comfortable during the procedure. If there is a chance that cancer has spread to the lungs, your doctor may perform a small lung biopsy during bronchoscopy.

Treatment

No symptoms

Pneumonitis that doesn't cause symptoms but can be seen on imaging tests is considered mild. Your doctor may recommend briefly pausing immunotherapy until a repeat chest CT (with contrast) is done. You will likely have a follow-up visit in 1 to 2 weeks to see if there is improvement.

Mild or moderate symptoms

Symptoms of pneumonitis include shortness of breath, cough, fever, and chest pain. If you have symptoms, immunotherapy will be paused. You will have some or all of the tests previously described. Until infection has been ruled out, you may be prescribed an antibiotic. Treatment with steroids will be started. Your doctor will check your symptoms and oxygen saturation about every 3 to 7 days.

Bronchoalveolar lavage

During a bronchoscopy, a small amount of sterile saline (saltwater) may be put into the lungs. The saline washes the airway and is then suctioned back through the tube. The fluid is tested for infection.

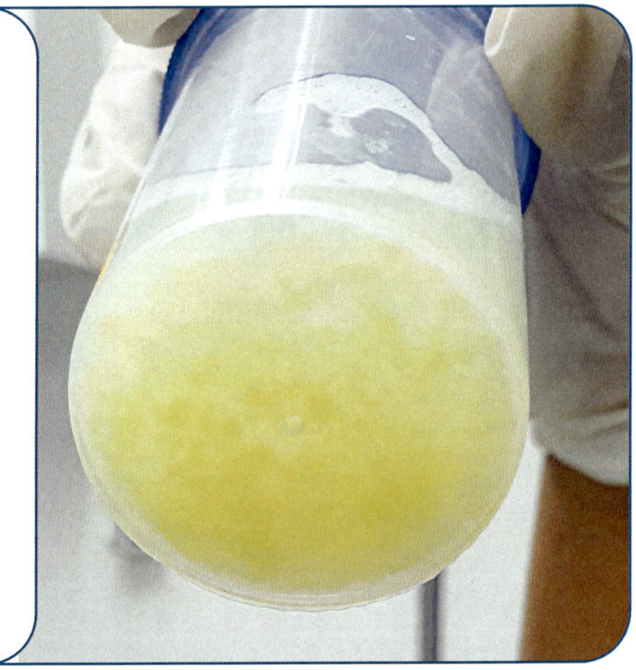

Severe or life-threatening symptoms

Pneumonitis is considered severe if you need extra oxygen to breathe and your symptoms are preventing basic self-care.

You will be admitted to the hospital for testing and monitoring. Immunotherapy will be stopped. Until infection has been ruled out, you may be prescribed an antibiotic. To rule out heart problems as the cause of your symptoms, a cardiologist (heart expert) may evaluate you.

Intravenous steroids will be started. If there is no improvement within 48 hours, treatment with one of the following may be added:

- Intravenous infliximab
- Intravenous immunoglobulin (IVIG)
- Mycophenolate mofetil

Key points

- Symptoms of inflamed lungs (pneumonitis) include trouble breathing, dry cough, fever, and chest pain.
- Testing for infection often includes a nasal swab to detect viruses and testing of your mucus, blood, and urine.
- Other testing may include bronchoscopy with bronchoalveolar lavage and a chest CT.
- Mild pneumonitis can be seen on imaging tests but does not cause symptoms. Immunotherapy can often be continued.
- Steroid therapy is needed for pneumonitis that is causing symptoms. Immunotherapy will be paused until symptoms are gone.
- For severe or life-threatening pneumonitis, in-hospital care and treatment with intravenous steroids is needed. Immunotherapy will be stopped.

7
Muscles and joints

Immunotherapy can cause joints, tendons, ligaments, bones, and muscles to become inflamed. This chapter describes these side effects and their treatment.

Blood tests can provide helpful information about muscle and joint problems. Your provider will order blood tests based on the suspected problem. Tests often ordered for these conditions include:

- C-reactive protein (CRP)
- Erythrocyte sedimentation rate (ESR)
- Rheumatoid factor (RF)
- Antinuclear antibodies (ANA)
- Anti-cyclic citrullinated peptide (anti-CCP)
- Comprehensive metabolic panel (CMP)
- Creatine kinase (CK) and aldolase
- Troponin (a protein found in heart muscle)

Inflammatory arthritis

Inflammatory arthritis is not a single disease. It is a group of disorders caused by immune attack on joints. Major types include:

- Rheumatoid arthritis
- Psoriatic arthritis
- Lupus
- Gout

Inflammatory arthritis is not the same as osteoarthritis, which is caused by use of a joint over many years. Also, inflammatory arthritis often affects joints throughout the body, rather than just one or two. Symptoms include:

- Joint pain
- Joint swelling
- Stiffness in the morning
- Stiffness after rest that improves with activity

Your doctor will examine the painful or swollen joints to see how they function. In addition to blood tests, you may have imaging of the affected joints. Your provider may also consult with a specialist in arthritis and similar conditions (a rheumatologist).

Options for treating inflammatory arthritis are described next. Severe arthritis can lead to permanent joint damage. If your symptoms are disrupting your daily habits and imaging tests show joint erosion, immunotherapy may be paused.

NSAIDs

If only 1 joint is affected or if pain is mild, nonsteroidal anti-inflammatory drugs (NSAIDs) are used to help relieve symptoms. Ibuprofen (Advil), aspirin, and naproxen (Aleve) are NSAIDs. Your provider may suggest treatment with celecoxib (Celebrex). It is a newer type of NSAID called a COX2 inhibitor.

Oral steroids

For more severe symptoms, you will be prescribed an oral steroid. If your symptoms haven't improved in 2 weeks, the steroid dose will be increased. If still no improvement, treatment with a DMARD (described next) will be considered.

DMARDs

Disease-modifying anti-rheumatic drugs (DMARDs) reduce the signs and symptoms of rheumatoid arthritis and can slow tissue damage. DMARDs include methotrexate, sulfasalazine, leflunomide (Arava), and hydroxychloroquine. Blood tests are needed to see if you are eligible for a DMARD.

Biologics

In some cases, treatment with a biologic will be considered. Biologics are made in a lab from living cells. These protein-based drugs target specific parts of the immune system. They are given by injection or through a vein.

Other medications

For severe symptoms that haven't improved with other treatment, a TNF inhibitor or an IL-6 inhibitor may be considered. Infliximab (Remicade) is a TNF inhibitor. IL-6 inhibitors include tocilizumab (Actemra) and sarilumab (Kevzara).

Muscle weakness and pain

Immunotherapy can cause muscle weakness, called myositis. Myositis most often affects muscles in the neck, upper arms, shoulders, hips, and thighs. There may also be muscle pain (myalgia).

Muscle strength testing can help find nervous system problems that may be causing the weakness. Your doctor may also order electromyography (EMG) or MRI of the affected muscle(s). EMG measures muscle and nerve function.

For milder symptoms, you will be prescribed an oral steroid. You will have blood tests on a regular basis to check the levels of creatine kinase and aldolase.

For severe or life-threatening symptoms, immunotherapy will be paused. You will be admitted to the hospital. Treatment with intravenous steroids will be started. For symptoms that don't improve with steroids, treatment with one of the following may be added:

- a DMARD (such as methotrexate)
- intravenous immunoglobulin (IVIG)
- mycophenolate mofetil
- rituximab

If you have muscle pain, your doctor will make recommendations for treating or managing your pain.

Polymyalgia rheumatica

Polymyalgia rheumatica (PMR) is a disorder that causes muscle aches, pain, or stiffness. The shoulders and hips are most often affected. The symptoms often come on quickly and are worse in the morning.

Blood and lab tests are used to gather more information. If your provider suspects PMR based on your symptoms, you may have an ultrasound of your shoulders, hips, or both.

PMR is treated with oral steroids. If there is no improvement, your steroid dose may be increased and immunotherapy paused. If symptoms persist, treatment with a DMARD or an IL-6 inhibitor may be added. You may be referred to a specialist for further care.

When your symptoms are gone, steroids will be tapered over 6 to 12 weeks (maybe longer).

PMR is closely related to another condition called giant cell arteritis, described next. Many people who have one of these also have symptoms of the other.

Polymyalgia rheumatica causes muscle aches, pain, or stiffness, especially in the shoulders. In addition to blood tests, you may have an ultrasound of your shoulders, hips, or both if this problem is suspected.

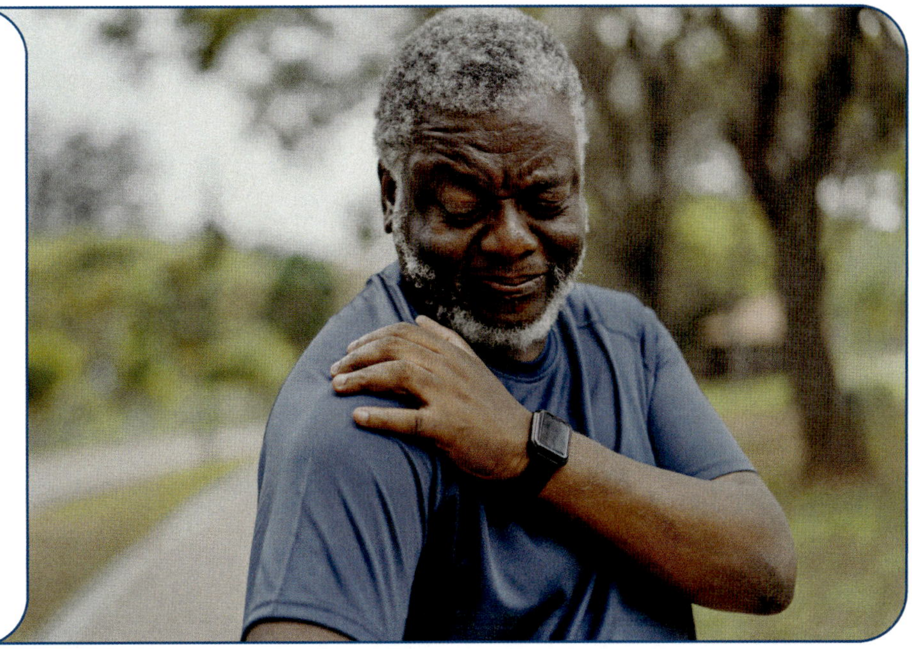

Giant cell arteritis

In giant cell arteritis (GCA), blood vessels on the sides of the forehead (the temporal arteries) become inflamed and more narrow. Symptoms include:

- Changes in eyesight
- Headaches
- Scalp tenderness
- Jaw pain from chewing or speaking
- Fevers, night sweats, and weight loss

If left untreated, GCA can lead to blindness. Your provider will refer you to a specialist right away for a temporal artery biopsy. In this procedure a tiny piece of scalp artery is removed for testing. The artery may also be examined using ultrasound. If GCA is confirmed, immunotherapy will be paused.

If you have vision changes, you will be referred right away to an ophthalmologist or vascular surgeon.

Giant cell arteritis is treated with oral steroids, and sometimes an IL-6 inhibitor. A rheumatologist will decide if an IL-6 inhibitor (such as tocilizumab or sarilumab) is a good option for you.

When your symptoms are gone, steroid therapy will be tapered extra slowly. The tapering period for GCA is at least 8 to 12 weeks.

Key points

- Inflammatory arthritis is a group of joint disorders. Symptoms include joint pain, joint swelling, and stiffness after rest. NSAIDs can relieve mild arthritis symptoms. If symptoms are more severe, oral steroids or a DMARD may be needed.
- Immunotherapy can cause muscle weakness (myositis), especially in the muscles closest to the trunk. Oral steroids are given for milder symptoms. Severe symptoms require inpatient care and intravenous steroids.
- Polymyalgia rheumatica (PMR) causes muscle pain and stiffness, especially in the shoulders. Symptoms are worse in the morning. An ultrasound of the shoulders and hips can help diagnose PMR. Treatment with oral steroids is needed.
- Symptoms of giant cell arteritis (GCA) include vision changes, headaches, scalp tenderness, and jaw pain. If left untreated, GCA can lead to vision loss. Treatment includes oral steroids and possibly an IL-6 inhibitor.

8
Less common side effects

Immunotherapy can have less common but serious effects on the nervous system, heart, kidneys, eyes, and pancreas. This chapter describes these uncommon but possibly severe problems. Urgent testing is often needed.

Nervous system

Nervous system side effects of immunotherapy are rare but serious. They can affect the brain, spinal cord, and nerves throughout the body.

Testing includes blood tests and usually several of the following:

- Magnetic resonance imaging (MRI) of the brain and/or spine
- Electromyography (EMG) and nerve conduction studies (NCS)
- Lung function and breathing tests
- Heart function tests, such as an electrocardiogram (ECG)
- Lumbar puncture
- Electroencephalogram (EEG)

Testing helps rule out bacteria and viruses as the cause of your symptoms.

Myasthenia gravis

Myasthenia gravis is a disease that causes muscle weakness. Symptoms include:

- Droopy eyelids
- Double vision
- Problems swallowing
- Weak face muscles
- Weak breathing muscles
- Weakness in the arms and legs

This condition can worsen quickly. In-hospital treatment is required for severe cases, and is often recommended for milder cases. Immunotherapy will be paused. For milder symptoms, treatment with oral steroids and pyridostigmine is given. Pyridostigmine is a muscle strengthener that works by raising the levels of a chemical in the nervous system.

Severe myasthenia gravis is treated with intravenous steroids and either plasmapheresis or intravenous immunoglobulin (IVIG). If needed, treatment with rituximab may be added.

Guillain-Barré syndrome

This nerve problem causes weakness of the arms, legs, face, breathing muscles, and eye nerves. The first symptom is often pain in the lower back and thighs. In-hospital treatment is needed.

When caused by immunotherapy, Guillain-Barré syndrome (GBS) is treated with intravenous steroids and either IVIG or plasmapheresis. Gabapentin, pregabalin, or duloxetine are options for pain relief.

Non-infectious meningitis

The meninges are the thin layers of tissue that cover the brain and spinal cord. When they become inflamed, it is called meningitis. When not caused by infection, it is known as aseptic or non-infectious meningitis. Symptoms can include:

- Headache
- Sensitivity to light
- Neck stiffness
- Fever
- Nausea or vomiting

If you have symptoms of meningitis, immunotherapy will be paused. If your symptoms are limiting self-care, they are considered severe. In-hospital care is needed. Your provider may start you on intravenous antiviral medicine until infection has been ruled out. Once it has, your provider may recommend steroid therapy, or choose to closely monitor you without steroids.

Inflamed spinal cord

The spinal cord carries messages between the brain and nerves in the body. If it becomes inflamed, these messages are blocked. This is called transverse myelitis. It causes problems with sensation and nerve function.

Symptoms include pain, muscle weakness in the legs (sometimes the arms), and sensory problems. Bladder and bowel problems are also common. In-hospital care is needed. Treatment with IV steroids will be started. If your symptoms don't improve or get worse, IVIG or plasmapheresis may be added.

Inflamed brain

Immunotherapy can cause the brain to become inflamed. This rare side effect is called encephalitis. Symptoms range from mild confusion to serious brain function problems. **See Guide 3.**

Immunotherapy will be paused if you have symptoms. Symptoms are considered severe if they are making self-care difficult. In-hospital care is needed for encephalitis that is severe or worse. Your provider may start you on intravenous antiviral medicine until infection has been ruled out. Once it has, treatment with intravenous steroids will be started. If steroids are not enough, either IVIG or plasmapheresis will be added.

If there is no improvement in 1 to 2 weeks, or if your blood has a specific protein, treatment with rituximab might be an option.

Guide 3 Encephalitis symptoms
Confusion
Changes in behavior
Headaches
Seizures
Short-term memory loss
Problems reacting or responding
Trouble speaking

Heart and blood vessels

Heart and blood vessel side effects are rare, but can come on quickly and become very severe.

Myocarditis

The heart muscle may become inflamed. This is called myocarditis. The heart becomes bigger (swollen) and weaker. Severe cases can lead to heart failure and changes in heartbeat. In people not on immunotherapy, myocarditis is usually caused by infection.

Symptoms include:

- Fatigue
- Chest pain or pressure
- Very slow, very fast, or irregular heartbeat
- Shortness of breath
- Swollen legs, ankles, or feet
- Lightheadedness

If you have symptoms you will be examined by a heart expert (cardiologist or cardio-oncologist). You will have testing to look for heart and blood vessel problems. The goal is to find heart problems early and learn if they are due to immunotherapy or other heart or blood vessel diseases. You may be admitted to the hospital for closer monitoring, for more testing, or for treatment.

Myocarditis is treated first with high-dose IV steroids. If there is improvement, you will be switched to oral steroids. Steroids will then be slowly stopped (tapered) and replaced with other medicines. During steroid tapering you will be monitored very closely. The goal is to reverse immune attack against the heart muscle, support and recover heart function, and prevent the myocarditis from recurring.

Damage to the heart muscle can lead to changes in heartbeat. Electrical defibrillation treatment and/or a pacemaker may be needed. This small device is implanted in the chest. It helps the heart to function. It may be needed permanently.

Other heart and blood vessel problems

The outer lining of the heart (pericardium) can become inflamed. This is called pericarditis. Fluid can build up around the heart (pericardial effusion) and may need to be removed.

Inflammation of blood vessels (arteries and veins) is also possible. This is called vasculitis.

Eyes

A number of symptoms can signal an eye-related side effect. **See Guide 4.**

If you have symptoms or vision changes, your doctor will refer you to an ophthalmologist for a complete eye exam. This eye expert will guide your care. Certain infections and diseases can cause eye problems. Your provider will order blood tests to rule out these and other possible causes of your symptoms.

Over-the-counter eye drops (artificial tears) can help with dryness and irritation. These saline (salt)-based drops moisturize and soothe the eyes. Contact lenses and eye makeup can make symptoms worse. Try to avoid these and other irritants.

Steroid eye drops are often all that is needed for mild symptoms. More severe symptoms may require steroids and pausing immunotherapy.

Uveitis

The layer of tissue beneath the white of the eye is called the uvea. It has 3 parts. When any of these parts is inflamed, it is called uveitis. If not treated, serious problems such as blindness can occur.

The part of the uvea that most often becomes inflamed is the iris. This is the colored ring around the pupil. Immunotherapy will be paused for iritis (also called anterior uveitis). Treatment with steroid drops is recommended. An oral steroid may also be prescribed.

Inflammation of the back of the uvea or of all three parts is less common. It is also more serious. Immunotherapy may be paused. Treatment with steroid eye drops, steroid eye injections, or an oral steroid is recommended.

Episcleritis

The episclera is a thin layer of clear tissue that covers the white of your eye. If this layer becomes inflamed it doesn't usually affect eyesight. Treatment is not always needed. Artificial tears can help with symptoms. immunotherapy is typically continued for mild inflammation. If there are changes in eyesight, immunotherapy may be paused. Treatment

Guide 4 Eye and vision symptoms
Blurred/distorted vision
Blind spots
Change in color vision
Sensitivity to light
Tenderness or pain
Eyelid swelling
Bulging eyes
Red or purple discoloration of the eye
New floaters
Itchy eyes
Eye redness

may include NSAID eye drops, steroid eye drops, or an oral steroid.

Scleritis

The sclera is the white of the eye. It protects the eye and helps maintain its structure. When the sclera is inflamed it is often painful. Other symptoms include eye tenderness, redness, and swelling.

Scleritis is considered mild if it does not affect vision. Mild scleritis is treated with an oral NSAID. Systemic (oral or intravenous) steroids are needed for scleritis that is causing vision changes. Immunotherapy may be paused.

Keratitis

The clear tissue on the front of the eye (the cornea) can also become inflamed. This is called keratitis. It does not usually affect eyesight. Treatment is not always needed. If the inflammation is mild, immunotherapy is typically continued. Artificial tears can help with symptoms.

If there are changes in eyesight, immunotherapy may be paused. Treatment may include steroid eye drops, an oral steroid, or a topical antibiotic.

Maculopathy

Maculopathy is damage to the center part of the retina, called the macula. It causes blurry central vision. Central vision is important. It's what you use to read, drive, and recognize faces. Immunotherapy will be paused, even for mild symptoms. Treatment for maculopathy may include steroid eye drops or an oral steroid.

If you have symptoms or vision changes, your doctor will refer you to an ophthalmologist for a complete eye and vision exam. Examination with a microscope with a bright light (a slit lamp) is a key part of a complete exam.

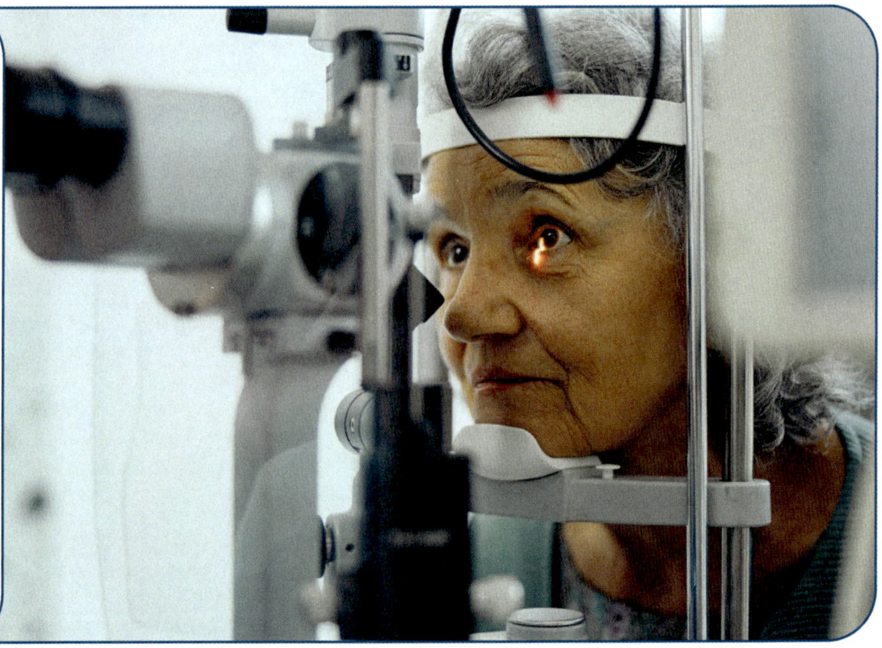

Kidneys

The kidneys remove waste and extra water from blood. One substance that gets filtered out is creatinine, a waste product of muscles. The level of creatinine in your blood and protein in your urine will be checked during immunotherapy. A high level of creatinine signals that the kidneys aren't working well.

Causes other than immunotherapy will be considered. Certain medicines can damage the kidneys if taken at a high dose for a long time. Your doctor will review your medications and make any needed changes.

Acute kidney injury

Acute kidney injury occurs when the kidneys suddenly stop filtering blood. This kidney crisis comes on quickly, usually in less than a few days. Wastes build up and disrupt blood's chemical makeup. Symptoms include:

- Making less urine
- Swollen legs, ankles, or feet
- Shortness of breath
- Fatigue
- Confusion
- Nausea
- Chest pain or pressure

In severe cases, seizures or coma are possible. In-hospital care may be needed. Treatment with steroids will be started. You may first have a kidney biopsy. Immunotherapy will be paused.

Pancreas

The pancreas does more than make hormones. It also makes substances that help digest food. These are called enzymes. When inflamed or injured, liver cells leak more enzymes than normal into the bloodstream.

Blood tests are used to check enzyme levels during immunotherapy. If the levels go up a little, any symptoms are usually mild and may include:

- Nausea
- Bloating
- Burping
- Pain in abdomen
- Back pain

No treatment is needed.

High levels, however, signal that the pancreas is under immune attack. It becomes very inflamed over a very short period of time. This is called acute pancreatitis.

If this is suspected, imaging with CT and sometimes a special type of MRI will be ordered. If confirmed, in-hospital care is needed. Treatment involves oral or intravenous steroids and intravenous fluids.

Key points

- Immunotherapy can cause rare but serious problems affecting the nervous system, heart, kidneys, eyes, and pancreas.
- Symptoms of a nervous system side effect can include muscle weakness, confusion, headaches, sensitivity to light, changes in behavior, and seizures.
- Heart and blood vessel side effects are rare but serious. Symptoms include worsening fatigue, chest pressure or pain, shortness of breath, heartbeat changes, and swelling in the lower body.
- Eye changes during immunotherapy can include dryness, pain, tenderness, redness, swelling, and vision changes. An ophthalmologist will guide your care.
- Symptoms of acute kidney injury include making less urine, lower body swelling, shortness of breath, fatigue, confusion, and nausea.
- High levels of substances made by the pancreas can be a sign of acute pancreatitis. This rare side effect requires in-hospital care.

Immunotherapy side effects can start even after treatment is over. Stay alert for new symptoms for at least 1 year after finishing immunotherapy.

9 Resources

Websites

AIM at Melanoma
aimatmelanoma.org

AIM at Skin Cancer
AIMatSkinCancer.org

Be the Match
BeTheMatch.org/one-on-one

CancerCare
Cancercare.org

National Coalition for Cancer Survivorship
canceradvocacy.org

The Leukemia & Lymphoma Society
LLS.org/PatientSupport

Triage Cancer
triagecancer.org

When to contact your cancer care team

✓ If you develop signs and symptoms, such as:

- Severe fatigue
- Headache
- Rash
- Cough
- Shortness of breath
- Chest pain
- Abdominal bloating
- Change in bowel habits
- Weight loss
- Vision changes or eye pain
- Severe muscle weakness
- Severe muscle or joint pains
- Mood changes

✓ If you are seen by a new health care provider

✓ If you are prescribed any new medication

✓ If you are admitted to the hospital

✓ Before getting any immunizations or vaccinations

Questions to ask

It is common to have questions for your care team about immunotherapy. Below are some that may be helpful.

1. Which immune checkpoint inhibitor(s) am I taking?
2. Which side effects does this regimen most often cause?
3. What is the best way to contact you (my care team) with a new symptom or concern?
4. Can I do it online?
5. Which symptoms should I report right away?
6. I forgot to take my steroid. What should I do?
7. I have questions about lowering my steroid dose. Who should I ask?
8. What can I do about my fatigue?
9. Can you give me an immunotherapy wallet card?

Words to know

aseptic meningitis
Inflammation of the tissues covering the brain and spinal cord that is not caused by a bacterial infection.

blister
A fluid-filled sac in the outer layer of skin. A medical emergency, especially when the mouth or genitals are affected.

colitis
Inflamed bowel (colon). A common side effect of immunotherapy.

corticosteroids
Lab-made drugs that slow the immune system. A common treatment for immunotherapy side effects. Also called steroids.

CTLA-4
A protein found on T cells that helps keep the body's immune responses in check. The immune checkpoint inhibitor ipilimumab is used to block CTLA-4.

diabetic ketoacidosis (DKA)
A diabetic emergency. Occurs when blood sugar drops dangerously low. Toxic acids (ketones) collect in the blood and urine.

diarrhea
Frequent and possibly watery bowel movements. A common side effect of immunotherapy.

encephalitis
Inflammation of the brain. A rare side effect of immunotherapy.

episcleritis
Inflammation of the thin outer layer of the eye. A rare side effect of immunotherapy.

giant cell arteritis (GCA)
Inflammation of the lining of the arteries, especially the arteries in the temples.

Guillain-Barré syndrome (GBS)
A rare condition in which the body's immune system attacks the nerves located outside the brain and spinal cord.

hepatitis
Inflamed liver. Does not often cause symptoms.

hypothyroidism
A condition in which the thyroid gland does not make enough thyroid hormone. Also called underactive thyroid.

immune checkpoint inhibitor (ICI)
A type of cancer treatment that blocks contact between immune cells and cancer cells. The most common type of immunotherapy.

immune-related adverse event (irAE)
A side effect of cancer immunotherapy.

inflammatory arthritis
A group of disorders caused by immune attack on joints. Includes rheumatoid and psoriatic arthritis.

intravenous immunoglobulin (IVIG)
Intravenous infusion of helpful antibodies collected from many donors.

maculopapular rash
A rash with both flat patches and bumps. A common side effect of immunotherapy.

myalgias
Pain in a muscle or group of muscles.

myasthenia gravis
A disease that causes weakness in the arms and legs, vision problems, and drooping eyelids or head.

myocarditis
A rare but severe immunotherapy side effect in which the heart muscle becomes inflamed. The heart may also become enlarged, weak, and abnormal heartbeat may occur.

myositis
Weakness, swelling, and/or pain due to inflamed muscles.

nonsteroidal anti-inflammatory drug (NSAID)
A drug that decreases fever, swelling, pain, and redness.

pancreatitis (acute)
Inflamed pancreas. A rare side effect of immunotherapy.

pericardial effusion
The buildup of fluid around the heart.

pericarditis
A condition in which the outer lining of the heart becomes inflamed. Can cause pericardial effusion.

pneumonitis
Inflammation of one or both lungs. The most common symptom is trouble breathing.

polymyalgia rheumatica (PMR)
A disorder that causes muscle pain and stiffness, especially in the shoulders.

pruritus
Itchy skin, with or without a rash. A common side effect of checkpoint inhibitors.

thyroiditis
Painless injury to the thyroid gland caused by immune attack. Causes thyroid hormone levels to rise temporarily before dropping too low.

transverse myelitis
A nervous system disorder in which both sides of one section of the spinal cord are inflamed.

uveitis
Inflammation of all or part of the middle layer of the wall of the eye (uvea). A rare immunotherapy side effect.

vasculitis
Inflammation of blood vessels (arteries and veins).

NCCN Contributors

This patient guide is based on the NCCN Clinical Practice Guidelines in Oncology (NCCN Guidelines®) for Management of Immunotherapy-Related Toxicities, Version 1.2024. It was adapted, reviewed, and published with help from the following people:

Dorothy A. Shead, MS
Senior Director
Patient Information Operations

Erin Vidic, MA
Senior Medical Writer, Patient Information

Susan Kidney
Senior Graphic Design Specialist

The NCCN Guidelines® for Management of Immunotherapy-Related Toxicities, Version 1.2024 were developed by the following NCCN Panel Members:

*John A. Thompson, MD/Chair
Fred Hutchinson Cancer Center

Bryan J. Schneider, MD/Vice-Chair
University of Michigan Rogel Cancer Center

Julie Brahmer, MD, MSc/Vice-Chair
The Sidney Kimmel Comprehensive Cancer Center at Johns Hopkins

Mohammad Abu Zaid, MBBS
Indiana University Melvin and Bren Simon Comprehensive Cancer Center

Amaka Achufusi, MD
University of Wisconsin Carbone Cancer Center

Philippe Armand, MD, PhD
Dana-Farber/Brigham and Women's Cancer Center | Mass General Cancer Center

*Meghan K. Berkenstock, MD
The Sidney Kimmel Comprehensive Cancer Center at Johns Hopkins

*Bonnie Bermas, MD
UT Southwestern Simmons Comprehensive Cancer Center

Tawnie Braaten, MD
Huntsman Cancer Institute at the University of Utah

Lihua E. Budde, MD, PhD
City of Hope National Medical Center

Saurin Chokshi, MD
St. Jude Children's Research Hospital/ The University of Tennessee Health Science Center

*Marianne Davies, DNP, RN, ACNP-BC, AOCNP
Yale Cancer Center/Smilow Cancer Hospital

Changchun Deng, MD
Case Comprehensive Cancer Center/ University Hospitals Seidman Cancer Center and Cleveland Clinic Taussig Cancer Institute

*Yaron Gesthalter, MD
UCSF Helen Diller Family Comprehensive Cancer Center

Michael Jain, MD, PhD
Moffitt Cancer Center

Prantesh Jain, MD
Roswell Park Comprehensive Cancer Center

*Benjamin H. Kaffenberger, MD, MS
The Ohio State University Comprehensive Cancer Center - James Cancer Hospital and Solove Research Institute

*Maya Khalil, MD
O'Neal Comprehensive Cancer Center at UAB

Melissa G. Lechner, MD, PhD
UCLA Jonsson Comprehensive Cancer Center

Tianhong Li, MD, PhD
UC Davis Comprehensive Cancer Center

Alissa Marr, MD
Fred & Pamela Buffett Cancer Center

Suzanne McGettigan, MSN, CRNP, AOCN
Abramson Cancer Center at the University of Pennsylvania

Jordan McPherson, PharmD, BCOP, MS
Huntsman Cancer Institute at the University of Utah

Theresa Medina, MD
University of Colorado Cancer Center

*Nisha A. Mohindra, MD
Robert H. Lurie Comprehensive Cancer Center of Northwestern University

Anthony J. Olszanski, MD, RPh
Fox Chase Cancer Center

Olalekan Oluwole, MBBS, MPH
Vanderbilt-Ingram Cancer Center

*Sandip P. Patel, MD
UC San Diego Moores Cancer Center

Jason Prosek, MD
The Ohio State University Comprehensive Cancer Center - James Cancer Hospital and Solove Research Institute

Sunil Reddy, MD
Stanford Cancer Institute

Pankti Reid, MD, MPH
The UChicago Medicine Comprehensive Cancer Center

*John Ryan, MBA
Patient Advocate

*Mabel Ryder, MD
Mayo Clinic Comprehensive Cancer Center

Bianca Santomasso, MD, PhD
Memorial Sloan Kettering Cancer Center

Scott Shofer, MD, PhD
Duke Cancer Institute

Jeffrey A. Sosman, MD
Robert H. Lurie Comprehensive Cancer Center of Northwestern University

*Yinghong Wang, MD, PhD
The University of Texas MD Anderson Cancer Center

Vlad G. Zaha, MD, PhD
UT Southwestern Simmons Comprehensive Cancer Center

Stephen Zucker, MD
Dana-Farber/Brigham and Women's Cancer Center | Mass General Cancer Center

NCCN Staff

Ajibola Awotiwon, MBBS, MSc
Guidelines Layout Specialist

Lisa Hang, PhD
Oncology Scientist/Senior Medical Writer

* Reviewed this patient guide. For disclosures, visit NCCN.org/disclosures.

NCCN Cancer Centers

Abramson Cancer Center
at the University of Pennsylvania
Philadelphia, Pennsylvania
800.789.7366 • pennmedicine.org/cancer

Case Comprehensive Cancer Center/
University Hospitals Seidman Cancer Center and
Cleveland Clinic Taussig Cancer Institute
Cleveland, Ohio
UH Seidman Cancer Center
800.641.2422 • uhhospitals.org/services/cancer-services
CC Taussig Cancer Institute
866.223.8100 • my.clevelandclinic.org/departments/cancer
Case CCC
216.844.8797 • case.edu/cancer

City of Hope National Medical Center
Duarte, California
800.826.4673 • cityofhope.org

Dana-Farber/Brigham and Women's Cancer Center |
Mass General Cancer Center
Boston, Massachusetts
877.442.3324 • youhaveus.org
617.726.5130 • massgeneral.org/cancer-center

Duke Cancer Institute
Durham, North Carolina
888.275.3853 • dukecancerinstitute.org

Fox Chase Cancer Center
Philadelphia, Pennsylvania
888.369.2427 • foxchase.org

Fred & Pamela Buffett Cancer Center
Omaha, Nebraska
402.559.5600 • unmc.edu/cancercenter

Fred Hutchinson Cancer Center
Seattle, Washington
206.667.5000 • fredhutch.org

Huntsman Cancer Institute at the University of Utah
Salt Lake City, Utah
800.824.2073 • healthcare.utah.edu/huntsmancancerinstitute

Indiana University Melvin and Bren Simon
Comprehensive Cancer Center
Indianapolis, Indiana
888.600.4822 • www.cancer.iu.edu

Mayo Clinic Comprehensive Cancer Center
Phoenix/Scottsdale, Arizona
Jacksonville, Florida
Rochester, Minnesota
480.301.8000 • Arizona
904.953.0853 • Florida
507.538.3270 • Minnesota
mayoclinic.org/cancercenter

Memorial Sloan Kettering Cancer Center
New York, New York
800.525.2225 • mskcc.org

Moffitt Cancer Center
Tampa, Florida
888.663.3488 • moffitt.org

O'Neal Comprehensive Cancer Center at UAB
Birmingham, Alabama
800.822.0933 • uab.edu/onealcancercenter

Robert H. Lurie Comprehensive Cancer Center
of Northwestern University
Chicago, Illinois
866.587.4322 • cancer.northwestern.edu

Roswell Park Comprehensive Cancer Center
Buffalo, New York
877.275.7724 • roswellpark.org

Siteman Cancer Center at Barnes-Jewish Hospital
and Washington University School of Medicine
St. Louis, Missouri
800.600.3606 • siteman.wustl.edu

St. Jude Children's Research Hospital/
The University of Tennessee Health Science Center
Memphis, Tennessee
866.278.5833 • stjude.org
901.448.5500 • uthsc.edu

Stanford Cancer Institute
Stanford, California
877.668.7535 • cancer.stanford.edu

The Ohio State University Comprehensive Cancer Center -
James Cancer Hospital and Solove Research Institute
Columbus, Ohio
800.293.5066 • cancer.osu.edu

The Sidney Kimmel Comprehensive
Cancer Center at Johns Hopkins
Baltimore, Maryland
410.955.8964
www.hopkinskimmelcancercenter.org

The UChicago Medicine Comprehensive Cancer Center
Chicago, Illinois
773.702.1000 • uchicagomedicine.org/cancer

The University of Texas MD Anderson Cancer Center
Houston, Texas
844.269.5922 • mdanderson.org

UC Davis Comprehensive Cancer Center
Sacramento, California
916.734.5959 • 800.770.9261
health.ucdavis.edu/cancer

UC San Diego Moores Cancer Center
La Jolla, California
858.822.6100 • cancer.ucsd.edu

UCLA Jonsson Comprehensive Cancer Center
Los Angeles, California
310.825.5268 • uclahealth.org/cancer

UCSF Helen Diller Family
Comprehensive Cancer Center
San Francisco, California
800.689.8273 • cancer.ucsf.edu

University of Colorado Cancer Center
Aurora, Colorado
720.848.0300 • coloradocancercenter.org

University of Michigan Rogel Cancer Center
Ann Arbor, Michigan
800.865.1125 • rogelcancercenter.org

University of Wisconsin Carbone Cancer Center
Madison, Wisconsin
608.265.1700 • uwhealth.org/cancer

UT Southwestern Simmons
Comprehensive Cancer Center
Dallas, Texas
214.648.3111 • utsouthwestern.edu/simmons

Vanderbilt-Ingram Cancer Center
Nashville, Tennessee
877.936.8422 • vicc.org

Yale Cancer Center/Smilow Cancer Hospital
New Haven, Connecticut
855.4.SMILOW • yalecancercenter.org

We want your feedback!

Our goal is to provide helpful and easy-to-understand information on cancer.

Take our survey to let us know what we got right and what we could do better.

NCCN.org/patients/feedback

Index

Made in the USA
Monee, IL
25 June 2025

19603567R00036